Jo H. Linsley

Handbook of uroscopy

Jo H. Linsley

Handbook of uroscopy

ISBN/EAN: 9783742819024

Manufactured in Europe, USA, Canada, Australia, Japa

Cover: Foto ©Lupo / pixelio.de

Manufactured and distributed by brebook publishing software
(www.brebook.com)

Jo H. Linsley

Handbook of uroscopy

→⚜ U R O S C O P Y ⚜←

FROM NOTES TAKEN IN THE LABORATORY OF

Jo H. Linsley, M. D.,

—— BY ——

SUMNER GLEASØN

STENOGRAPHER,

BURLINGTON,　　　--　　　　--　　　VERMONT.

R. S. Styles, Printer, Burlington, Vt.

PHYSICAL PROPERTIES.

CHAPTER I.

The Urine is the typical excretion of the body. It is the product of change of animal tissue, and is excreted from the Malpighian bodies and convoluted tubes of the kidney. The kidneys have nothing to do themselves with the formation of the urinary principle; they simply purify the blood by separating the effete matters, and the urine is simply a solution of urea and chloride of sodium with more or less of the organic and inorganic constituents of the blood.

If normal urine is allowed to stand uncovered for a while, a small cloud of mucus sinks to the bottom of the vessel.

It is claimed that there is an acid and an alkaline fermentation of the urine. The acid fermentation is thought to be due to the decomposition of the extractive coloring matter by the vesical mucus, producing lactic and acetic acids. The alkaline fermentation which takes place after the acid fermentation is due to the decomposition of urea. At this time you get the granules of urate of ammonium and microscopic crystals of urate of sodium. The acid fermentation of the urine is however doubted.

The following names are given to the urine according to the hour in which it is passed:

Urina Sanguinis, the urine that is first passed in the morning. It has a specific gravity of 1015 to 1025 or 1030.

Urina Potus, that passed after large quantities of water have been taken. Specific gravity of 1002 to 1015.

Urina Cibi, the urine of digestion ; which has a specific gravity of 1020 to 1030.

Urina Spastica, the urine of disease.

QUANTITY. The quantity of urine in 24 hours is from 40 to 52 ounces, or from 1200 to 1600 c. c. The most urine is passed in the afternoon, less in the morning, and least of all at night.

The quantity of urine is increased *normally* by repose, exposure to cold, dry skin, unusual imbibition, taking of food, after eating fruit, in winter, use of stimulants, diuretics, alkalies, salines, and by certain drugs as cantharides, opium, and belladonna.

It is increased *pathologically* in convulsions, in acute diseases, after nervous attacks as hysteria, and in both forms of diabetes.

It is diminished *normally* by the use of diaphoretics, or anything that will increase perspiration, and by the administration of drastics.

It is dimished *pathologically* in diseases producing anarsarca and dropsy, suppression, uræmia, fevers, diarrhœa, nephritis, scarlatina, later stages of cardiac disorders, stage of collapse in cholera, all forms of Bright's disease except in the cirrhotic and lardaceous kidney.

COLOR. The normal color of urine is a yellow with more or less admixture of red.

The coloring matters are not definitely known, but later we shall consider two normal coloring matters of the urine, namely Urobilin and Indican.

The urine first passed in the morning is the darkest, and that passed in the forenoon the palest.

The color of course is subject to great variation in disease. The color table of Neubauer & Vogel is the one now used to determine the color of the urine by. It is composed of three sets of colors, pale urines, high colored urines, and the dark urines.

A pale urine long continued indicates a certain degree of anæmia, if the *amount* is normal. You get an almost colorless urine in the neuroses; and in a granular kidney the coloring matters are lost.

Blood red, or high colored urines, are a dark yellow with tendency to flame red, and they generally depend upon the presence of Urocrythrine, an abnormal coloring matter present in fever. They are generally concentrated, have a large amount of solids, are acid, and contain a large percent of urea.

The blood red, or garnet-red urines, are always caused by foreign coloring matters, as blood, etc. The dark urines are from diseases of the kidneys producing hæmorrhage, also by passage of biliary coloring matters. In leprosy near death, the urine becomes a dark brown. It is a dark red during the course of the disease.

Green urine of a dirty hue, comes from jaundice caused by the presence of Biliverdin, and it has the same significance as brown icteric urine.

We get a dirty blue urine in cholera and typhus fever, and at the same time we generally have a dark blue color to the skin. This urine has an alkaline reaction.

Blood coloring matters may be from a doubtful origin. They may be excreted from the kidneys, or they may have arisen by the breaking down of the blood corpuscles in the urine. If from hæmorrhage of large vessels, the urine contains mostly hæmoglobin and is red. If from capillary hæmorrhage, the urine contains mostly methæmoglobin, and has a brown color. The reason is, in capillary hæmorrhage the blood mixes with the urine slowly and is held longer in solution at the normal temperature of the body.

The temperature, carbonic acid in the urine, and want of oxygen, furnish the necessary conditions for the change from hæmoglobin to methæmoglobin.

Hæmaturia occurs in constitutional diseases such as scrofula, purpura, and scarlatina.

Then the urine may be of a muddy, brownish yellow color, from the presence of pus in cystitis, pyelitis, urethritis, gonorrhœa, abcess or suppuration of the bladder, prostate, or the urinary passages.

Iron, logwood, carbolic acid, and tar give the urine a black color when absorbed into the system. Santonin, a yellow or brownish red. Rhubarb, senna, or hæmatoxylon give a reddish color, and this is distinguished from bile by the addition of liquor ammonia, which turns the vegetable coloring matter to crimson. Tannin taken by the mouth renders the urine colorless.

An acid added to the urine after the taking of rhubarb or senna turns them a brighter color, and if it were blood it would be turned darker.

Odor. The cause of the normal odor of urine is unknown. It is described as *"urinous"*, or simply aromatic. Albuminous urine of a low specific gravity is almost odorless. Most alkaline urines give off an ammoniacal odor.

Saccharine urine gives a sweet whey-like odor. Some phosphatic urines give an excessively fetid odor. The odor is strong in rheumatism, gout, acid indigestion, and catarrh of the bladder. This is intensified by the addition of strong acids. After ingestion turpentine gives an odor of violets. Asparagus, copaiba, cubebs, sandal wood oil, garlic, saffron, and cauliflower, each give an odor to the urine peculiar to the substance taken.

In paraplegia, the urine has a fetid odor soon after passing.

CONSISTENCE. As to the consistency of the urine, it is a limpid fluid; never anything else in health but aqueous, dropping and flowing readily. Pathologically it is viscid, glutinous, and divided into drops with difficulty. This may be due to an excess of pus or mucus, as in acute catarrh. It may be a mixture of pus and mucus, and may also be due to the action of an alkali on pus or albumen.

The froth of normal urine readily disappears. If it is permanent, albumen, sugar, or bile pigments may be suspected.

SPECIFIC GRAVITY. The specific gravity of the urine may be normally from 1005 to 1028, with an average of 1020. It is always heavier than water.

The specific gravity is reckoned by comparison with distilled water. There are three ways in which it is obtained. First by the picnometer or specific gravity bottle, second by the urinometer or spindle, and third by the Mohr-Westphal balance. The temperature in all should be 60 degrees F., or 15 degrees C.

If the amount of urine be too small to use the spindle, add four volumes of water. Take the specific gravity and multiply excess over a thousand by 5 and add 1000.

Example. Suppose after adding four volumes the specific gravity is 1003; then 3 times 5 equals 15, plus 1000 equals 1015, the specific gravity of the urine.

In taking the specific gravity, a "stand test tube" should be used and the urine poured in at an obtuse angle, and the tube filled three-quarters full. The urinometer should then be introduced and the tube filled "to the brim." The specific gravity should be read where the *upper* surface of the urine cuts the scale on the urinometer.

The spindle should be gently touched on the end, causing it to descend to the bottom of the tube and back. This prevents any adhesions there might be between the sides of the tube and urinometer.

The specific gravity is high in diabetes mellitus, rheumatism, gout, fevers, after prolonged exercise, after excessive perspiration, and the first stage of acute Bright's disease.

It is low in albuminuria, pneumonia, in dilute urine, diabetes insipidus, after hysteria, in all forms of Bright's disease except acute nephritis.

Where there is an obstruction of the ureter by calculi passing, the characteristics of the urine passed will be that it is small in quantity, pale in color, and of a low specific gravity.

SOLID MATTERS. The normal amount of solid matters in the urine is from 60 to 80 grams. May be determined by multiplying the last two figures of the specific gravity by either the coefficient of Trapp, (which is 2) or of Haser, (2.33). Multiplying by either of these coefficients gives the number of grams of solid matters in 1000 c. c. or a litre of urine. If solids amount to 200 grams, look for sugar. If 20 grams, and the quantity *not correspondingly diminished*, hydruria or watery urine.

In fevers where the patients fast, 30 grams would be an average. If in pneumonia you have 40 grams upon a strict diet, the solids are increased at the expense of the tissues of the body.

Urea and chloride of sodium are the principal normal solid matters of the urine. In 100 parts of solid matters, there are 50 of urea, 25 of chloride of sodium, and the other salts of the urine make up the remaining 25.

REACTION. The reaction of urine is normally faintly acid. It is due to the acid phosphate of sodium and potassium. It may be normally neutral or faintly alkaline.

If the urine is alkaline, it should be determined whether this alkalinity occurred before or after being voided. If a sample of urine is alkaline when examined, it should be ascertained whether this is due to a fixed, (sodium or potassium compounds) or to a volatile alkali (ammonia). This is determined by gently heating and drying the red litmus paper turned blue by the presence of an alkali. If when dry the red color returns, the alkalinity is due to a volatile alkali. If the blue color is permanent, it is due to sodium and potassium compounds. If due to sodium and potassium compounds, nothing pathological is indicated. If due to ammonia when passed, it indicates an inflammation somewhere along the genito-urinary tract, causing an increased amount of mucus and of course with the decomposition of urea.

The urine is strongly acid in rheumatism, gout, acid indigestion, after taking hot and highly nitrogenous stimulating articles of food, and alcohol.

The urine may be alkaline normally in the middle of the forenoon, after a full meal, and after eating fruit. Pathologically in severe forms of paraplegia, in cystitis, retention of urine, and when pus is present. It can be made alkaline by the ingestion of the carbonates, acetates, citrates, or tartrates of the alkalies.

NORMAL CONSTITUENTS.

CHAPTER II.

UREA.

Urea, (CON_2H_4) is the product of oxidation of the nitrogenous substances of the body. The average is 35 grams in 24 hours. This may be in health considerably diminished or increased. It is found normally in the blood, bile, liver, amniotic fluid, vitreous and aqueous humors, and sweat. Not found in the muscle of man. It is soluble in water and alcohol. Insoluble in ether

Urea exercises more influence on the specific gravity than any of the other normal constituents of the urine. In fact its weight is equal to the entire weight of the other normal constituents. Unless a fluid contain urea, it is not urine.

The amount is *increased* after an animal diet, relatively in children though not absolute, during waking hours, in fevers up to the acme of the disease, and after, diminished below normal.

The amount is *diminished* when urea is retained in the animal economy, on vegetable diet, toward the fatal termination of disease, Bright's disease, at night, and in strong ammoniacal urine.

In diabetes mellitus if much sugar be present, the urea is diminished in per cent., though the total quantity in 24 hours is increased.

TEST. Take two samples of the urine and evaporate one sample to one-half the quantity, and then bring a drop of this in contact with a drop of nitric acid on a glass slide. If crystals of nitrate of urea do not form immediately, urea is diminished. Take a drop of the sample that is not evaporated and bring it in contact with a drop of nitric acid, and if crystals of nitrate of urea form immediately after adding, the urea is increased.

The amount of urea can readily be determined by comparison, in the absence of sugar or albumen. For instance, we have a specific gravity of 1025 normally. If the chlorides are found to be normal, then *urea* will be said to be normal, because there can be nothing else normally besides urea that will make up this amount of solids, the other salts exerting but very little influence on the specific gravity.

CHLORIDES.

The *chlorides* found in the urine are principally the chlorides of sodium and potassium. There is also ammonium chloride and possibly calcium chloride. The average is 14.73 grams in 24 hours.

The secretion of the chlorides is greatest in the afternoon and least at night. They are increased at first by drinking water, and later on, diminished ; are increased with a liberal salt diet and with energetic bodily or mental exercise. Increased during the paroxysms of intermittent fever, and the day after they are diminished. Also diminished in acute rheumatism. Increased in diabetes insipidus, in dropsy when diuresis comes on, febrile diseases when there are any serous exudations or watery discharge, in chronic affections accompanied by impaired digestion. They are said to be entirely absent from the urine during the height of pneumonia, and their reappearance is a sympton of improvement in the patient's condition. When not found in the urine, they are found in some of the other secretions, as the saliva. The amount seemingly depends upon the digestive powers of the patient.

TEST. First add a drop or two of nitric acid to hold the phosphates in solution. Then add two or three drops of a solution of nitrate of silver, and if normal the chlorides are thrown down as a white curdy precipitate.

The ability to calculate the normality or abnormality of the different normal ingredients of the urine by qualitative analysis, can only be learned accurately by experience.

THE EARTHY AND ALKALINE PHOSPHATES.

The *earthy phosphates* are the phosphates of calcium and magnesium. Average amount is from 1 to 1½ grams in the 24 hours.

The amount of magnesium phosphate is double that of the calcium phosphate. If the acid magnesium phosphate is acted on by ammonia, an ammonium magnesium phosphate is formed.

The earthy phosphates are *increased* in diseases of bones, especially when diffuse, as diffuse periostitis, rachitis, and arthritis. Also diseases of nerve centers, after great mental strain, after use of mineral waters rich in carbonates, and with exclusive meat diet, though not constant.

They are *diminished* in kidney difficulties.

TEST. Hoffmann and Ultzmann. A test tube, 16 cen-

timeters long, 2 centimeters wide, is filled one-third full
with clear or filtered urine.   Add a few drops of liquor potassa or ammonium hydrate, and warm until the earthy
phosphates separate out as a floculent precipitate.   After
setting aside for 10 or 15 minutes to settle, we can approxi-
mately estimate the amount.   If the layer of earthy phosphates is 1 centimeter high, the phosphates are normal.   If
the layer is 2 or 3 centimeters high, the earthy phosphates
are increased.   If on the contrary only single flakes appear,
then they are diminished.

The *alkaline phosphates* are the acid sodium phosphate
and possibly the potassium phosphate.   They average from
2 to 4 grams in the 24 hours.

The monophosphate of sodium, $(PO_4H_2NA,)$ causes acid
reaction of the urine more than any other.

The acid phosphate of sodium, $(PO_4HNA_2,)$ and neutral
phosphate of sodium, $(PO_4NA_3,)$ are alkaline in reaction.

The amount is influenced by the food.   They are quite
soluble in water and alkaline fluids.   Two-thirds of all the
phosphoric acid is in combination with the alkalies.

The alkaline phosphates are increased by inflammation
and fevers.

Both forms of phosphates if deposited in the urine indi-
cate an alkaline reaction, and are favorable to the formation
of phosphatic calculi.

TEST.   To a small quantity of urine in a test tube, add
about one-third of the magnesium mixture.   If the precipitate present a whitish granular appearance, the alkaline
phosphates are normal.   If on the contrary the color ap-
proaches a milky appearance, they are increased.   On the
other hand if only a slight precipitate is noticed, then they
are diminished.

Phosphoric Acid.

The amount of phophoric acid is from 2.3 to 3.8 grams in 24 hours. Average, 2.8 grams.

It is *increased* after the ingestion of phosphorus or the phosphates, after a principally meat diet, with common febrile disease, though not constant.

It is *diminished* in urines of low specific gravity, in the urina potus and spastica, kidney and heart diseases with less amount of urine, severe disorders of digestion, all chronic diseases of the brain except epilepsy.

In the urine, phosphoric acid, or orthophosphoric acid is combined with the alkaline earths.

Sulphates.

The *sulphates* are principally of sodium and potassium, sulphate of sodium being the most abundant. The average amount in 24 hours is from 2 to 2.1 grams. They are mostly influenced by the food.

They are greatest during digestion, and are increased upon drinking water, decreased after. Pure sulphur increases them and also a meat diet. They are increased in acute febrile processes, with a large excretion of urea. The greatest increase is noticed in meningitis, enchephalitis, rheumatism, and affections of the muscular system causing waste of tissue.

They are diminished with exclusive vegetable diet, in beginning of typhus fever, and (in per cent.) in all urines of a low specific gravity.

Their increase or decrease is not of great account in disease.

TEST.   As a solution of chloride of barium added to the urine precipitates the *phosphate* of barium (as well as the sulphate,) we add a drop or two of hydrochloric acid to a small quantity of urine in a test tube, and then one-third as much of the chloride of barium solution as we have urine to be tested.   If the sulphates are normal, we observe a milky appearance.   If the sulphates are increased, this is more of a creamy consistency; and if diminished, on the other hand, the color is lighter.

COLORING MATTERS.

The coloring matters are not definitely settled.   Urobilin and indican will be considered as the normal coloring matters of the urine.

UROBILIN.

It is supposed to be a reduction product of the coloring matter of the bile, bilirubin, though it is more likely to be the product of hæmoglobin. · Urobilin is the same substance which is spoken of in different works as urophain, urohæmatin, and urochrome.   A pale urine may contain much urobilin.   It is especially abundant in high colored urines of fevers.

TEST.   Pour a layer of pure sulphuric acid into a small beaker, then pour on this from the height of about ten inches twice as much urine.   If urobilin is normal, a deep garnet red color will be observed.   If increased, the color will be darker and opaque; and if diminished, of course lighter.

INDICAN.

Indican is the same as the uroxathon of Heller, and indigogen of Thudichum.

Pathological Significance. Increased by an exclusively meat diet, in Addison's disease, cholera, carcinoma of liver and stomach, in all diseases which threaten closure of the small intestine, (though not so much so in stoppage of the large intestine), peritonitis, chlorosis, in chronic diseases, inanition and cirrhosis of the liver, pyelitis, and diseases of the spinal cord.

Certain drugs, as turpentine, nux vomica, and the oil of bitter almonds, also increase it.

TEST. To a little pure hydrochloric acid in a test tube, (about 6 cubic centimeters) add 5 or 6 drops of the urine to be tested. Heat, and if the color is a pale yellowish red, indican is present in normal amount. If it turn a purple or violet color, it is increased.

URIC ACID.

Uric Acid, ($C_5 N_4 H_4 O_3$), is a less oxidized stage of urea, and is only found as a sediment when the urine is very acid. It is found in the urine of all classes of animals ; occurs even in the very lowest orders ; in the excrement of birds, snails, reptiles, and insects ; is found normally in the blood of hens. It is constantly increased in the blood in gout. Has also been found in the spleen, lung tissue, and gouty deposits. Its quantity is not so much dependent upon food as urea. It is soluble with difficulty in cold water, but more readily soluble in warm. Is generally found combined in the urine with its salts, as with the urates.

It is *increased* by indigestion, poor nutrition, in most

febrile conditions, more especially with disorders of the respiratory organs and disturbances of the circulation, rich animal diet, by too little exercise in open air, acute febrile processes which cause much breaking down of the nitrogenized elements of the body, in lung and heart diseases where there is dyspnœa, where the diaphragm is impeded in its function as by large tumors in the abdominal cavity, and by impoverished blood.

It is *diminished* in chronic affections of the kidneys, sometimes in diabetes mellitus, in hydruria, arthritis, and during paroxysms of gout.

MUREXID TEST. When present in the urine as a precipitate, we filter the urine and dry the filter, and then collect the sediment in a porcelain capsule. Add a few drops of nitric acid and warm carefully until dissolved ; then evaporate slowly with great care to near dryness and add a drop or two of ammonium hydrate. If uric acid is present, we get a purple red color, (murexid acid, or purpurate of ammonia.)

If a drop of a solution of nitrate of silver in the cold be brought in contact with a drop of a solution of uric acid, you have a brownish yellow or black spot, according to the amount of uric acid present.

To obtain uric acid from the urine, add one part of hydrochloric acid to eight parts of the urine, set aside for 24 hours and collect as above stated.

URATES.

The *urates* are salts of uric acid. They are the urates of sodium, potassium, ammonium, calcium and magnesium. Urate of sodium is the most common. Ammonium next. They are soluble at the temperature of the body and in alkaline solution. Are generally deposited during fevers, after copious perspiration. A precipitate of them is favored by concentration of the urine either by adding uric acid or by taking away the water, by the cooling of the urine, and by moderate acidity of it. If the urine is strongly acid, it throws down the uric acid instead of the urates.

TEST.—The urates are the only deposit found in the urine which clear up on the application of heat.

MUCUS.

There is always present in the urine a small quantity of mucus. This may be seen in time by allowing the urine to settle in a beaker, when the mucus will be observed as a little cloud floating below the middle of the liquid. It may be present in considerable quantities and still not to be seen owing to the transparency. If there is no color, and if there be a large quantity of mucus suspected, color the urine and then precipitate the mucus by alcohol which has some tincture of iodine in it. May also be precipitated by acetic acid with iodine in solution with potassium iodide. Urine containing much mucus filters badly. It is increased principally from irritation from the urinary tract. As a rule there is a larger amount in the urine in females than in that of males. Mucus may be separated from the urine by filtration, when it will be seen on the filter as a glistening coat of varnish.

OTHER NORMAL CONSTITUENTS OF THE URINE.

Creatine, Creatinine, Xanthin, Hippuric Acid, Oxalic acid, Lactic and Phenylic acids, are also normal constituents of the urine, but will not be here spoken of.

ABNORMAL CONSTITUENTS.

CHAPTER III.

ALBUMEN.

Albumen is the most important substance which the body requires for its preservation. It is the chief constituent of the blood, lymph, chyle, serous fluids, and the liquids of the cellular tissue. It is found in the urine after the use of egg albumen. Serum albumen may appear in very small quantities (from one to one-tenth per cent.) in the urine of a man healthy to all appearances, without serious consequences. What causes this is not known. The urine thus discharged is concentrated very highly, strongly acid, and contains a large quantity of urea and also uric acid. The reason why albumen is *not* found in the normal urine, is because it penetrates animal membranes with difficulty, and only under great pressure, unless there be destruction of the urinary tubules.

It is found in the urine pathologically when the blood pressure is greater than normal, in heart disease or impeded venous circulation, and most frequently in those affections of the kidney which are classed under the head of Bright's disease ; or in other words, those diseases which involve an alteration of the diffusion membrane of the kidney. The Royal College of Physicians of London include all diseases of the kidney productive of albuminuria as Bright's disease, and these are nephritis, nephritis albuminosa, inflammation of the malpighian bodies, granular kidney, cachectic nephritis, tubal nephritis, amyloid diseases of the kidney, etc. It is found, too, if blood, pus, or other albuminous fluid is mixed in the urine. This condition is termed false albuminuria. Also, it is sometimes found where there is imperfect nutrition of the capillary wall. This is termed hydraemia.

. TESTS.—Heat and the nitric acid tests are the only two responsible tests for the determination of the presence of albumen in the urine.

Take a small quantity of the urine in a test tube, if not acid, acidulate carefully with one or two drops of acetic acid, and heat. *Nitric* acid if added might form with the albumen an acid albuminate which would not be precipitated on the application of heat. Also, if an alkali was added in excess, an alkali albuminate would be formed and again the albumen would not be precipitated upon heating the urine. If a cloudiness occur after the urine is boiled for a few seconds it may be the earthy phosphates or albumen. Add a drop or two of nitric acid. If the cloudiness disappear, it is due to the earthy phosphates, and if it is still present albumen is found.

NITRIC ACID, OR HELLER'S TEST. Fill a test tube to about half an inch with pure nitric acid. Float carefully upon this a layer of urine to be tested. If a white ring be formed between the two liquids, it may be either albumen, the urates, or a resinous substance found in the urine after the ingestion of copaiba or oil of turpentine. To distinguish between albumen and the urates, we heat the liquid. If this ring clears up, it is due to the urates ; if not to albumen or the resin. To determine whether it be this substance (found in the urine from the ingestion of the above medicines) or albumen, add a few drops of alcohol. If it clear up, it is due to the substance above referred to. If *not*, if the ring is still present on the application of the above tests, we are *positive* albumen is in the urine.

When sulphuric acid is added to albumen, we get a violet color.

Concentrated nitric acid with heat gives a yellow color, then the addition of sodic hydrate gives an orange red color.

Also, most of the metallic salts as mercuric chloride and alum precipitate albumen.

Application of Trommer's test gives a violet color.

SUGAR.

Grape sugar is identical with diabetic sugar.

Sugar is found normally in the contents of the small intestine, chyle, after taking food containing sugar or starch, in the hen's egg both in the process of hatching and in those not being hatched, in the yolk as well as the white, in the amniotic and allantois fluid of cows, sheep and swine, and in the liver. There is no sugar in the urine normally.

When it is present in diabetes mellitus, it is also present in the blood and vomited matters, saliva, sweat, etc. Sugar is sometimes found temporarily in certain diseases. Also found in disturbances of the abdominal circulation, in convulsions, from some acute diseases especially cholera, when there are carbuncles, after severe burns, typhus fever, sometimes in rheumatic fever, and acute encephalitis. By wounding certain points of the medulla in animals, sugar is temporarily present in the urine.

Many diabetic urines have an odor somewhat like chloroform.

TESTS. *Moore's or Heller's Test.* Take two volumes of urine and one volume of liquor potassa in a test tube, and boil. If sugar is present, we observe a color varying from a pale red to a deep wine color, according to the amount of sugar present.

Böettger's Test. Add to a small quantity of urine in a test tube, a few drops of a solution of carbonate of soda. Then add a pinch of the sub-nitrate of bismuth, and heat. If sugar is present, we get a black precipitate of metallic bismuth. Albumen if present must be removed by precipitation by heat and then filtration, as if present will also give a black precipitate. The sulphur compounds will give a black precipitate. To distinguish whether it be due to sugar or the last named compounds, we add to the urine a small quantity of a solution of acetate of lead, and if the precipitate is due to the sulphur compounds, we have here a black precipitate. You may use instead of bismuth, litharge (or oxide of lead,) which will only be turned black by the sugar.

Trommer's Test. Add to a small quantity of urine in a test tube from 3 to 5 drops of a solution of sulphate of copper, and then an equal volume of liquor potassa, and heat. If sugar is present we get a red precipitate of the sub-oxide of copper.

A precipitate somewhat similar to this is occasionally observed in the urine of a healthy person by the coloration of the earthy phosphates. If this mistake is liable to occur the urine should be decolorized by shaking up with animal charcoal and filtering, when the test may be applied as given.

Fehling's Test. Mix one volume of No. 1 and two volumes of No. 2, dilute with about 50 or 60 c.c. of distilled water. To a small quantity of this in a test tube, add an equal quantity of urine and heat.

If sugar is present, we observe the same reaction as we had in Trommer's test.

Mülder's Test. (Indigo.) We add to a small quantity of urine in a test tube 2 or 3 drops of a solution of indigo, then render the reaction neutral or alkaline, by the addition of a solution of sodium carbonate, and heat without shaking. If sugar is present, the blue color disappears and we have a pale yellow color. Upon shaking the urine in contact with air, the blue color may be returned. (The indigo solution is made by rubbing up common indigo with Nordhausen sulphuric acid.)

Fermentation Test. Take three test tubes, fill the first with the urine to be tested, the second with a solution of glucose, and the third with water. Invert the three below the surface of some water. Under each place a small piece of German yeast, and allow to stand in a room with a temperature of about 60 to 70 degrees F. for 12 to 24 hours. At the end of this time, if some gas be observed in the number one and number two, and none in number three, sugar is present. If it be observed in number two and not in number one and number three, there is no sugar in the urine. If there be gas in all three, the yeast is worthless, and the test must be repeated with reliable yeast.

Piffard's Cupro-Potassic Paste. This is made of sulphate of copper, one part; crystallized Rochelle salts, five parts; caustic soda, c. p. two parts; rub up well in a mortar. To use, take a piece about the size of a pea, put into the test tube, add a little water and boil until dissolved. Then add a little urine, and if sugar is present we observe the precipitation of the sub-oxide of copper as in Trommer's test. This paste should be kept in a well stoppered vessel and put in a cool place.

From Neubauer & Vogel. Add to a small quantity of urine in a test tube a little weak ammoniacal solution of nitrate of silver, and boil for some time. If sugar be present, we will get a deposit of metallic silver in the form of a polished mirror on the bottom and sides of the test tube. The only other substance which will give this reaction with the above solution is tartaric acid.

Add to the urine a solution of caustic potassa, and then a few drops of the molybdate or tungstate of ammonia. Heat to boiling and then acidulate carefully with hydrochloric acid. You get a blue color if sugar be present.

If the urine be high colored with any of the above tests, it should be shaken up with animal charcoal and filtered. To do this, put one or two ounces of the urine in an eight ounce bottle, add half an ounce of charcoal and a small quantity of carbonate of soda. Shake well for from five to ten minutes, and filter. Then when ready to test, acidulate carefully with acetic acid.

UROERYTHRINE.

Uroerythrine is the coloring matter to which all high colored fever urines owe their color. It should contain iron. The presence of uroerythrine indicates the breaking down

of blood corpuscles during febrile processes. The foam of
urine containing much urocrythrine is yellow, and might be
mistaken for the foam of an icteric urine. To distinguish
it, add a little acetate of lead solution, when, if it be due to
bile, the precipitate will be yellow, while if due to urocrythrine it will be a flesh color or reddish. Urocrythrine occurs in all febrile conditions but most' frequently in
pyæmia, liver affections and lead colic.

TEST, by solution of acetate of lead. A solution of
acetate of lead added to the urine throws down all the coloring matters and some of the salts. The precipitate normally is white. If colored a pale flesh color or pinkish,
urocrythrine is present.

BILE.

There are tests for the biliary acids and for the biliary
coloring matters. As the biliary acids are found so rarely
in the urine, we shall not discuss them.

The coloring matters of the bile found in the urine are
bilirubin, biliverdin, biliprasin, and bilifuscin. These coloring matters are found, of course, in the bile, biliary calculi, intestine, and in the excrement. Pathologically, in
jaundice they are found in all the fluids of the body and
even pass into the tissues.

Detection. Urine containing them in large amount is
always strongly tinged a deep brown, reddish brown, greenish brown, dirty green, or grass green. It foams strongly,
and colors filter paper yellow or greenish.

GMELIN'S TEST. Put about an inch or so of concentrated
nitric acid which has been decomposed by standing in the
light, and carefully cover this with a layer of urine by

means of a pipette. If the coloring matters of the bile be present, we get a play of colors, a green ring which slowly rises, and on the lower border have finally a blue, violet, red, and yellow ring. Albumen in no wise interferes with the test.

A *better way* of conducting this test, is, by adding to a drop of urine in a porcelain capsule a drop of the above acid, when the play of colors will be better observed.

To biliverdin is due the green color.

HELLER'S TEST. Put in a test tube about 6 c.c. of pure hydrochloric acid, and then add enough urine drop by drop to distinctly color this. Allow 2 or 3 c. c. of pure nitric acid to flow down the side and underlie it. If biliary coloring matters are present, you have a play of colors.

The biliary coloring matters can also be detected by wetting a clean linen cloth or filter paper with the urine to be tested and allow it to dry. It is colored brown if biliary coloring matters be present.

BLOOD.

Blood may be found in the urine from disease of the kidney, disease of the pelvis or ureter, disease of the urethra, and in women from uterine discharges such as menstruation. If the amount of blood is large, it probably comes from the pelvis of the kidney, ureter, or bladder. If from the pelvis or ureter, generally pus or gravel is present.

Detection. If the urine is acid the corpuscles remain normal for some time, though generally swollen. Their color is generally palish, but more or less sharply defined. All these changes are caused by the water. Where the amount of blood is small, we allow the urine to stand for some little

time in a conical shaped vessel and the corpuscles will settle
to the bottom as a red sediment. This can be generally
recognized by the unaided eye as blood. The urine always
contains more or less albumen if blood is present.

TESTS. Add a little liquor potassa to the urine, heat to
boiling and allow the earthy phosphates which are separated by the alkali, to settle, when if blood be present,
they carry down the hæmatine and appear as a brownish
red, and sometimes as a very handsome blood red precipitate. If this red coloring matter were due to the coloring matter of plants, the phosphates during their precipitation would not carry with them any of the coloring
matter.

A few cubic centimeters of tincture of guiac is mixed
with an equal volume of oil of turpentine and shaken until
an emulsion is formed, when the urine is added carefully.
When this emulsion comes in contact with the urine, the
guiac resin is precipitated as a white, and later on as a dirty
green precipitate. If the urine contains blood, the resin is
colored more or less intensely blue. Urine containing albumen or pus does not give the above reaction.

To distinguish between the presence of blood and a red
color from the ingestion of some vegetable matters, we
add a little nitric acid. If it be due to blood, the color
is darker. If due to a vegetable coloring matter, it is
turned brighter.

Pus.

Pus when in the urine is more certainly recognized by
the use of the microscope. Pus settles quickly in an acid
urine when at rest.

Donné's Test. Pour the urine from the sediment, or extract the precipitate by means of a pipette, and to this add a little liquor potassa. If the substance be pus, it loses its white color and becomes a clear vitreous mass. And this has the consistence of the white of egg.

Pus may come from any part of the genito-urinary tract. If it comes from the pelvis of the kidney, it is less apt to be mixed with mucus, and the urine retains its normal reaction longer. Pus is readily mixed with the urine and is promptly deposited from it. From the bladder however, if the urine is not alkaline when voided, it is apt to become so very soon from the presence of a large quantity of mucus. In females you may get pus in the urine from leucorrhœa, etc.

VOLUMETRIC ANALYSIS.

CHAPTER IV.

UREA.

HYPOBROMITE TEST. Solution is made up with 100 grams of caustic soda ; 25 c. c. of bromine ; and 250 c. c. of distilled water.

The test depends upon the decomposition of urea by the above hypobromite solution ; nitrogen being given off is measured, and from the amount of nitrogen so disengaged is calculated the amount of urea in the quantity of urine used. (5 c. c.)

PROCESS. A tall glass cylinder, 22 inches high and 2 inches wide, is filled with water. In this a burette of 100 c. c. is inverted. A rubber tube connects the end of the burette with a mixing flask. (Any two ounce wide mouthed vial will answer the purpose.) The stopper of the mixing bottle flask has two holes in it ; through each of these a piece of glass tubing is put, to one is attached the tube from the burette and to the other a piece of tubing on which is a pinch cock. In the flask is placed 15 c.c. of the hypobromite solution. 5 c. c. of the urine is put in a small tube (a test tube broken off near the end answers the purpose very well) and carefully placed (*without mixing with the hypobromite solution*) in the bottle. The stopper is now placed in and pressed firmly in place, and the pinch cock closed. The reading on the burette is now taken and noted. The urine and the hypobromite solution are then allowed to mix, the flask being shaken up. They should be well shaken, and the decomposition allowed to continue for at least three-quarters of an hour, and during this time the surface within the burette should be kept at a evel with that on the outside. At the end of this time the reading is again taken. The difference between the two readings multiplied by .0027 gives the number of grams of urea in 5 c. c. of urine used. From this can be easily calculated the amount in the whole quantity.

The reason for multiplying by .0027, is that .0027 of a gram of urea when decomposed by the above solution gives off 1 c. c. by measure of nitrogen gas.

HYPOCHLORITE TEST. Take of Labarraque's solution, (liquor sodæ chlorinatæ, Squibb's) seven parts, and the urine one part. Get specific gravity of mixed solutions. After decomposition, which should take two hours, get the specific gravity. Subtract the specific gravity of the mixture before decomposition took place, and multiply the difference by .77, and you have the per cent. of urea. To get the specific gravity of the mixed urine before decomposition, multiply the specific gravity of the hypochlorite solution by 7, add the specific gravity of the urine and divide by 8. Ex. Suppose that of the hypochlorite solution is 1045 and that of the urine 1010, then 1045 by 7 plus 1010, divided by 8 = 1040—the specific gravity of the mixture before the reaction.

CHLORIDE OF SODIUM.

Standard solution required is made up by dissolving 14.53

grams of nitrate of silver in 1000 c. c. of distilled water. 20 c. c. of this solution equals one decigram of chloride of sodium.

A saturated solution of chromate of potash.

PROCESS. Put 100 c. c. of filtered urine in a beaker. Add four times as much distilled water with 2 or 3 drops of the chromate of potash solution. Render the reaction neutral or faintly alkaline by carbonate of soda or nitric acid, as the case requires. Bring the beaker under the burette filled to the 0 mark with the standard solution of nitrate of silver. Add in small quantities at a time until the last addition is followed by a permanent red appearance. Get the number of c. c. of nitrate of silver solution used and divide this by 20, and you have the number of grams of chloride of sodium per litre of urine.

We do this because the standard solution is made up so that 20 c. c. equal one decigram of chloride of sodium. Then dividing by 20 gives the number of decigrams of chloride of sodium in 100 c. c., and in 1000 c. c., or a litre, there would be ten times as much, or just so many grams instead of decigrams.

PHOSPHORIC ACID.

Standard Solution of Nitrate of Uranium. Dissolve 35.2 grams of nitrate of uranium in 1000 c. c. of distilled water. 20 c. c. of this solution equal one decigram of phosphoric acid.

Solution of Acetate of Sodium. Dissolve 50 grams of acetate of soda in 500 c. c. of distilled water and add 50 c.c. of acetic acid.

Solution of Ferrocyanide of Potassium, strength of one to ten.

PROCESS. Put 100 c. c. of urine in a beaker, add 25 c. c. of the solution of acetate of soda, a little water, and warm. Have a slip of white glass or a porcelain capsule handy on which is several drops of the ferrocyanide solution. When the mixture is warm, bring it under the burette filled with the standard solution of nitrate of uranium, and titrate carefully. When a drop from the beaker brought in contact with a drop of ferrocyanide strikes a brown color, the analysis is terminated, and the number of c. c. used divided by 20 will give the number of grams of phosphoric acid per litre of the urine.

SULPHURIC ACID.

Standard solution of barium chloride ; dissolve 15.25 grams of chloride of barium in 1000 c. c. of distilled water. 20 c. c. of the solution equals one decigram of sulphuric acid.

Solution of sulphate of soda, strength of one to ten.

PROCESS. Put 100 c. c. of urine in a beaker, add about 200 c. c. of distilled water, a little hydrochloric acid, and place the mixture in a water bath or hold over a spirit lamp until hot. Fill the burette to the 0 mark with the standard solution of barium chloride and bring the beaker under it. Permit a small portion of this solution to drop into the beaker and allow precipitate of sulphate of barium to settle. Continue addition carefully, allowing mixture to settle each time until there is a clear strata of fluid above. Then add a drop or two more of the barium chloride. If this causes a fresh precipitate continue carefully as before, but if no precipitate occurs, bring a drop of the clear fluid in contact with a drop of the solution of sulphate of soda :

if now a dense white precipitate appears, it shows too much chloride of barium has been added to the urine and the analysis must be repeated. The number of c.c. of standard solution finally determined on as necessary for the precipitation of all the sulphuric acid, divided by 20 will give the number of grams of sulphuric acid per litre of urine.

ALBUMEN.

Take 25 c. c. of the urine, acidulate carefully with acetic acid if not already acid, and heat until the albumen is all precipitated. Then filter this through a previously weighed dry filter. Place the filter with the precipitate upon it in a water oven and keep there until perfectly dry. Then allow it to cool in a desiccator and weigh. The difference between the weight of the filter before and after filtering gives the amount of albumen in 25 c.c. of urine. The amount of albumen in the 24 hours can then be readily calculated.

SUGAR.

Fehling's solutions consist of two solutions, No. 1 and No. 2.

Solution No 1. Made by dissolving 51.98 grams of c. p. sulphate of copper in 500 c. c. of distilled water.

Solution No. 2. 259.9 grams of Rochelle salts, c. p., dissolved in 1000 c. c. of a solution of caustic soda, c. p. of a specific gravity of 1.12.

PROCESS. Mix one volume of No. 1 with two volumes of No. 2. Put 20 c. c. of the mixed solution in a flask, dilute with 60 c. c. of distilled water, and boil. Dilute the urine with 4 volumes of water. Fill the burette to the 0 mark with the diluted urine. When the Fehling's solution boils, bring it under the burette and add the urine very carefully, a little at a time, until all the blue color is discharged and a faint red color is present. Then divide the number of c. c. used by 5 and the quotient is the number of c. c. of urine containing one decigram of sugar.

CHEMICALS AND APPARATUS.

CHAPTER V.

CHEMICALS.

CH. P. Nitric Acid.

CH. P. Hydrochloric Acid.

CH. P. Colorless Sulphuric Acid.

Pure Acetic Acid.

Liquor Potassa of the U. S. P.

Solution of Sodium Carbonate, one part of the crystalized salt to three parts water.

Solution of Barium Chloride, four parts crystalized barium chloride, sixteen of distilled water and one of hydrochloric acid.

Magnesian Mixture ; containing magnesium sulphate and ammonium chloride, each one part, distilled water eight parts, pure liquor ammonia one part.

Solution of Sulphate of Copper, ten grains to the ounce.

Solution of Nitrate of Silver, one part to eight of distilled water.

Solution of Acetate of Lead, one part to four of distilled water.

APPARATUS.

Half a dozen five inch. and half a dozen six inch test tubes.
A Test Tube, on foot.
Test Tube Rack and Drainer.
2 Conical Glasses.
Red and Blue Litmus Paper.
Filter Paper.
Urinometer, with a scale from 1000 to 1050 or 1060.
Spirit Lamp.
3 Porcelain Capsules.
2 Nests of Beakers, 3 each.
3 Glass Funnels.
Glass Stirring Rod.
Pipette.
1 Wash Bottle.
1 Test Tube Cleaner.

Set of 13 bottles with glass blown labels, of 4 ounce capacity, are preferable to any other. Care should be taken that the stoppers of the liquor potassa, barium chloride, magnesian mixture, acetate of lead, and carbonate of soda bottles are parafined.

For Volumetric Work.

Burette of 100 c.c. and one of 50 c.c. with float and pinch cock, and a clamp for burette.
Pipettes, one each of 100, 50, 25, 15, 10, and 5 c. c.
1 Litre Flask.
1 Graduated Cylinder, Stoppered, 500 c. c.
Sand Bath, Water Ovens, etc.

INDEX.